THE SEVEN STEPS TO NATURALLY STRONGER IMMUNITY

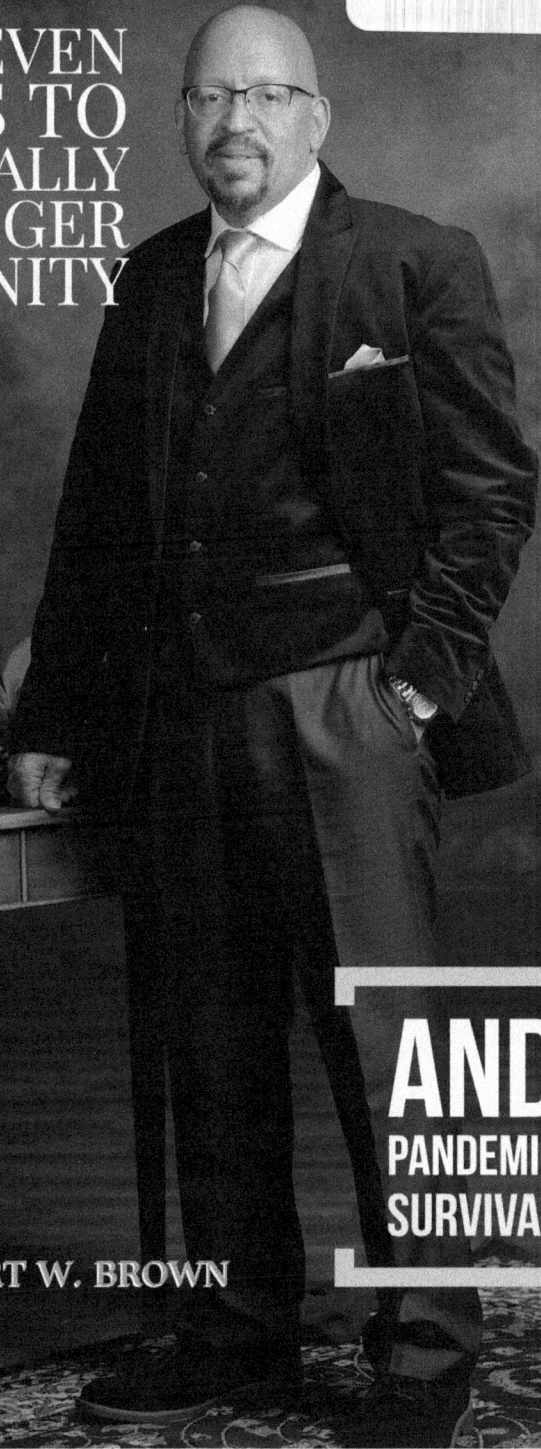

AND
PANDEMIC SURVIVAL

DR. STUART W. BROWN

THE SEVEN STEPS TO NATURALLY STRONGER IMMUNITY AND PANDEMIC SURVIVAL

DR. STUART W. BROWN

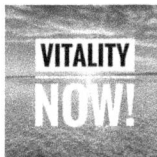

VITALITY
NOW!

I dedicate this book to all truth seekers who, despite all the chaos in the world today, remain rooted, grounded, and steadfast in whatever moral attitudes they were instructed, along with the necessary adjustments that they had to make along the way. More are coming.

CONTENTS

Foreword   ix
Preface   xi
Introduction   xiii

1. The Naturopathic Approach   1
2. STEP 1: TISSUE CLEANSING AND BOWEL   3
   MANAGEMENT
   Bowel Management   4
   Where It All Happens—The Small Intestine   5

3. STEP 2: ELIMINATE THE BAD STUFF   8
   Gluten   9
   Roundup (Glyphosate)   10
   Oils In A Bottle   12
   Fried Food   13
   How Trans Fat Harms You   14
   Burnt Animal Fat   16
   Baked Potato Skins   16
   Processed Meats   17
   Carbonated Beverages With A Meal   18

4. STEP 3: EAT HEALTHILY   20
   Carnivorous Considerations   22

5. STEP 4: MANAGE STRESS LEVELS   25
   Supplementation That May Help Fight Cytokine Storm   28

6. STEP 5: EXERCISE AND SLEEP   30
   Exercise   31
   Sleep   33

7. STEP 6: SUPPLEMENT WITH MEDICAL NUTRITION   35
   Lack of Nutrition In Foods   36
   Lack of Minerals   37
   Food Irradiation   38
   Though Nutritional Supplements Are Unregulated, They   38
   Are Generally Safer Than Prescription Drugs

FOREWORD

A truly revolutionary book! The contents of this work completely changed how I view nutrition. If you are looking for a book that can equip you to achieve excellent health, you've found it. Dr. Stu Brown taught me significant steps to take toward a healthy life, which revolutionized my knowledge of nutrition, and now this insight is available to everyone. Don't miss this book if you want to stay healthy. My inspiration and mentor has been Dr. Brown. I am one of the hundreds who have been impacted by his health knowledge. Having known Dr. Brown for over 15 years, I am completely overjoyed and enthused by his scholarship that I endorse and recommend this nutritional treasure.

Dr. Willie Dye
    Biblical Archaeologist'

PREFACE

I am Dr. Stuart W. Brown, the originator of the website VitalityNow-Health.com. My wife Cynthia and I are both disciples of Christ who believe in every promise made to God's people, as referenced in Genesis through Revelation. We also accept that our bodies are gifts to us, are the temple of the Holy Spirit, that we are not our own, and to quote the apostle Paul, "...no one ever hated their own body, but they feed and care for their body, just as Christ does the church--for we are members of his body." (Eph. 5:29) I also hold an Associate of Arts degree in Business Management, A Certificate of Achievement in TV and Film Editing, and a Doctor of Divinity from Bible Believer's Christian College and Seminary. I am not a medical doctor, and the medical advice I give here is only for reference. You should always consult with a medical practitioner in your local area when addressing any medical concerns.

The challenges of writing this book came after realizing that even though I was educating myself about health and wellness through over 25 years of independent research, I hadn't lived up to the standard. More specifically, in May of 2012, my blood glucose level was 419 mg/dL. To those who don't already know, normal fasting glucose levels should be between 66 – 99 mg/dL. Of course, when glucose in the blood becomes elevated for an extended length of time, it adversely affects other body processes. So, things like homocysteine, triglycerides, LDL cholesterol, and C-reactive protein became elevated. MDs call this condition metabolic syndrome, and its causes are obesity, diabetes or pre-diabetes, and mineral deficiencies.

Metabolic syndrome is like the red lights that go on in your car, warning you that something is wrong and needs attention. The lights warn the driver that whatever is not looked at soon could bring on significant trouble later. It doesn't mean that the car will immediately die. Metabolic syndrome consists of several preexisting conditions that, if not taken seriously, will bring failure to several of the body's systems.

At this point, I want to let you in on a little secret. Of the seven steps that I will deliver to you through this book's pages, your health during a pandemic requires you to take care of these warning lights. Elevated LDL cholesterol, obesity, hypertension, osteoporosis, atherosclerosis, pre-diabetes, and diabetes are warning lights that this book provides methods of battling naturally.

During my journey, not only did I learn that diabetes was nutrition-based, but I also discovered that so was arthritis, Alzheimer's, cancer, fibromyalgia, and a host of other degenerative diseases. I hope I can encourage you, whether you are presently under a doctor's care, or don't feel like your old self anymore, or want to stay on top of good health as you age and check out *The Mighty 90*. The Mighty 90 consists of 60 minerals, 16 vitamins, 12 amino acids, and two essential fatty acids, and they will make a drastic difference in the way you feel. You don't have to live out the last 10 or 20 years of your life being sick like your parents and grandparents did.

INTRODUCTION

These are the opinions that I share with Dr. Peter Glidden, ND, as being the root causes of our current medical system crisis.

1. When it comes to the treatment of chronic disease, MD directed pharmaceutical medicine doesn't work.

2. Most people only know about MD addressed pharmaceutical drugs because it is the only medical system that our hospitals provide, and our medical insurance covers.

3. The average person is hesitant and suspicious of anything other than MD directed medicine because the American Medical Association has successfully orchestrated a 100-year long slander and smear campaign against all of their "alternative" competitors. Anyone who is not an MD became labeled a quack (by the MDs), and consequently, outlaws their profession from the practice of medicine.

Increasing your immunity is a journey, not a destination. Having good health requires constant vigilance and maintenance that your body, soul, and spirit will reward you. If you are serious about improving your physical condition, accept that your body isn't like Amazon Prime, where you will receive the delivery of your results in two days. You have a lifetime accumulation of debris in your complex bodily systems that gained a footing over years of abuse, and now you will be embarking upon a journey to reverse the damage it caused. If you act with diligence, almost to the point of obsessiveness, you can change nearly any unfavorable condition with God's help and with the medical nutrition known to us today. If the same money and effort invested in the pharmaceutical industry in search of lucrative patents became available to naturopaths for research, we would have even more information on medical nutrition than we do today. Nevertheless, also if your condition is not better in 90 days, you will still be on a path to recovery and healing instead of a steady decline in health.

The steady decline to which I am referring is one that has Allopathic medicine at its core. *Iatrogenic* is a term that many people don't recognize. It is not a popular term among doctors because it points to their faults, yet it is the third leading cause of death. It ranks third behind heart disease and cancer. Iatrogenic is a Greek term that means "brought forth by the healer." What this means is the diagnosis or treatment of a physician had a negative result that often leads to the death of a patient. Think of one of the miracles of Jesus in the Gospels (Matthew 9:20–22, Mark 5:25–34, Luke 8:43–48), where there is a woman with an issue of blood. In Mark, the Scripture reveals that "And a woman was there who had been subject to bleeding for twelve years. She had suffered a great deal under the care of many doctors and had spent all she had, yet instead of getting better, she grew worse. MDs practice Allopathic medicine, which has no room for God. The absolute legalistic nature by which the practice exists precludes any type of faith or belief system when adhering to double-blind research studies. After administering all the surgeries, medicines, and radiation fail, the patient is placed "in God's hands." All this begs the question, "Wouldn't it have been wiser for the patient to have never left God's hands in the first place?" Unless the patient was the victim of a gunshot wound, fell off the roof of a house, or collided with a bus, most often, this type of intervention usually is not needed. On the other hand, Naturopathic medicine has a different approach, which is the one that we follow.

Before you heal someone, ask him if he is willing to give up the things that made him sick. — Hippocrates

---

Chapter One

THE NATUROPATHIC APPROACH

Naturopaths and Allopaths are on entirely different courses of action when it comes to reckoning with chronic illness. The Naturopathic approach is to benefit the body's natural mechanism of defense by encouraging its immune system to attack any foreign invaders. The Allopathic approach uses other foreign substances or methods (synthetic chemicals, drugs, radiation, or surgery) that suppress the body's natural immune response.

Allopathic medicine has a monopoly on health and wellness in general, which is supported by the present status quo. I also must mention that health care costs in this country are the leading cause of bankruptcy. Per person, the US spends about triple the expenditure on health care compared to every other industrialized nation in the world! Of all the industrialized countries in the world, the health of US citizens ranks second from the bottom. Unfortunately, most health insurance policies will not cover your costs if you decide to see anyone other than an MD for your health concerns. Medical treatments by Naturopaths support and promote the healthy function of the human body by design. The body's built-in self-healing mechanisms become stimulated using these methods. More often than not, the treatments delivered by Naturopaths help patients to recover from whatever illness they have been suffering ultimately. It's time to take back your health from the MDs and get to the root cause of your symptoms. Pain or discomfort is the signal your body is giving you that something is out of balance in your body's systems. Instead of only masking the pain or discomfort and further weakening your immune system as well as your bank account, let's aim for the cure.

Chapter Two

STEP 1: TISSUE CLEANSING AND BOWEL MANAGEMENT

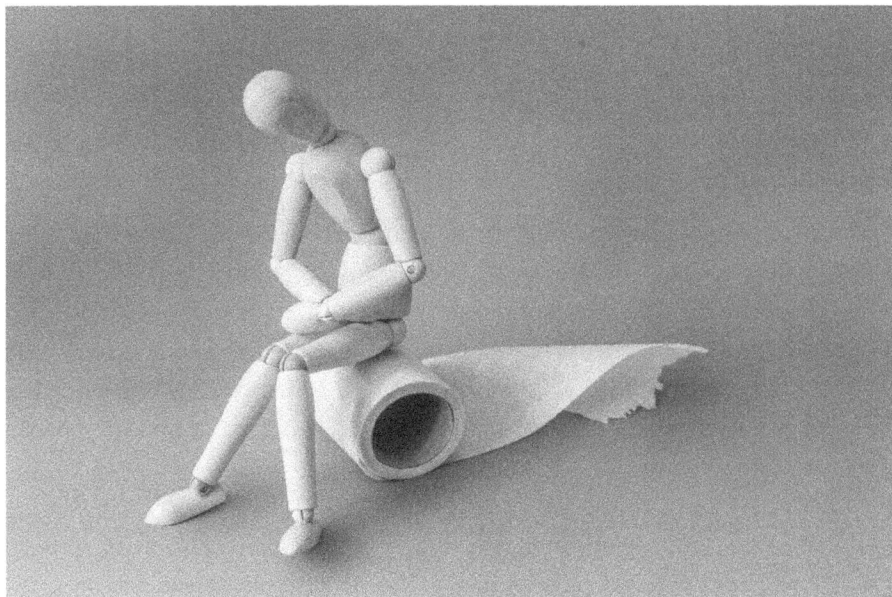

For I will restore health to you And heal you of your wounds,' says the Lord. Jeremiah 30:17

Most people, after they are sick, will pay large amounts of money to get well. What I have discovered is that you can't pay for good health, but you can earn it by working for it. A visit to the doctor for treatment of some sort may temporarily leave you feeling better, but unless you elevate your thinking, you will be right back where you started by going back to the same old habits. We all need to learn to manage our kitchens at home or else wind up again in the hospital where one operation can lead to another. The most crucial factor that affects immunity to sickness and disease is having a healthy bowel.

The importance of immune modulation at the gastrointestinal level can be understood easily, considering that approximately 70% of the entire immune system is found in this site and that in the lamina propria there are about 80% of all plasma cells responsible for IgA antibody production.[1]

BOWEL MANAGEMENT

The above-stated fact is where most people's health problems lie. Poor bowel management is at the root of poor health. Knowledge of a healthy bowel was much more prevalent 100 years ago, but somehow after Allopathic medicine gained a stronghold in 1901, the culture seemed to vanish into thin air. For example, it is more common today when we are dealing with poor bowel performance to visit CVS to purchase a laxative rather than taking an enema.

People have used enema solutions for centuries to treat constipation, bowel issues, and to cleanse their colon. But the benefits of enemas stretch even further in the body. Enemas help eliminate toxins that have been stored in the body. The benefits range from improving circulation, boosting energy, losing weight, clearing the skin, detoxing the liver, improving regularity, bowel cleansing, and more.[2]

WHERE IT ALL HAPPENS—THE SMALL INTESTINE

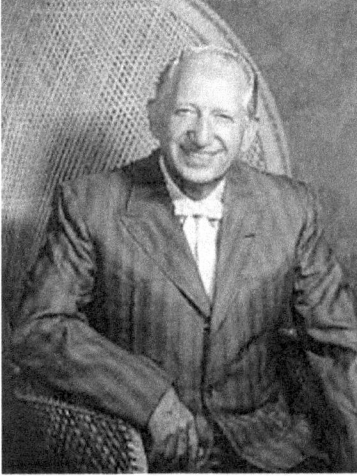

Dr. Bernard Jensen

In the center of the digestive tract lies a 5-foot tube referred to as the small intestine. The lining of this tube is adversely affected by chronic exposure to food toxins and allergens, which deteriorate its facing and expose the body to ailments, such as "leaky gut syndrome." The leaky gut syndrome is when microscopic food particles end up in the circulatory system due to a weakened intestinal wall. The root of chronic degenerative diseases that affect the heart, brain, respiratory tract, and bone and muscle activate the immune system and cause inflammation. The resulting continuous assaults draw upon the resources of the body's immune system to fight the offenders and induce healing. But if the assaults are ever-continuing, over time, the healing and repair will become suppressed. When this occurs, other bodily systems will be adversely affected, causing pain, swelling, cold symptoms, hypertension, and various organs behave dysfunctionally, paving the way for health to deteriorate gradually. If not corrected, it just keeps getting worse until a doctor can name it and start billing your insurance company for his or her treatment of it.

For The Life Of The Flesh Is In The Blood. Lev. 17:11

The circulatory system is the sacred space of the human body, and the Bible declares it in Leviticus 17:11. When microscopic food particles enter the bloodstream and circulate through the many organs of the body, they prompt a defensive reaction within the circulatory system itself. The defensive molecules of the circulatory system come into contact with the offending food particles within the various organs of the body, and disease symptoms begin.

As these blood scavengers go into attack mode against the invaders, the blood becomes "dirty." The lymphatic system shifts into high gear depositing lymphocytes with vital nutritional elements, particularly essential fatty vitamins (D, E, A, and K). Still, as the toxicity continues, they will become less available. The reason this happens is the same reason why the blood became dirty in the first place. Digestive system and food issues are to blame. These same undigested, microscopic food particles enter the lymph system directly via capillaries that line the intestine. If this only happens once or twice, it's OK, but if this is a chronic condition, it complicates things. When the lymphatic system becomes congested, beware of edema, weight gain, hypertension, respiratory problems, cancer, heart disease, and all kinds of immune and autoimmune disorders.

In the next section, I will discuss the biggest offender of the small intestine and how its elimination has the potential to change your life all by itself. To learn more about maintaining this all-important system of the body, I recommend reading Tissue Cleansing Through Bowel Management by Bernard Jensen, DC. Ph.D., Nutritionist. Considered the definitive work on the relationship of intestinal flora to tissue health, this enduring classic has sold over 1 million copies. Dr. Jensen's recommendations have motivated numbers of people to take responsibility for their health and well-being. His protocols have helped them find relief from numerous bowel- and tissue-related diseases.

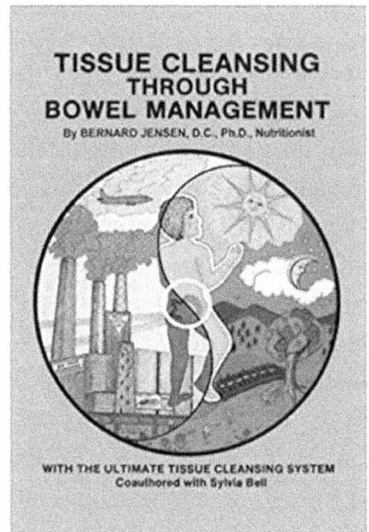

TISSUE CLEANSING THROUGH BOWEL MANAGEMENT
By BERNARD JENSEN, D.C., Ph.D., Nutritionist

WITH THE ULTIMATE TISSUE CLEANSING SYSTEM
Coauthored with Sylvia Bell

---

1. Vighi, G., et al., (2008) Allergy And The Gastrointestinal System. 153 Suppl 1(Suppl 1), 3–6. https://doi.org/10.1111/j.1365-2249.2008.03713.x

2. Asprey, D. (2020) 7 Best Enema Solutions To Cleanse And Detox Your Body (With Recipes) https://blog.daveasprey.com/enema-solutions-cleanse-detox-recipes/

Chapter Three

STEP 2: ELIMINATE THE BAD STUFF

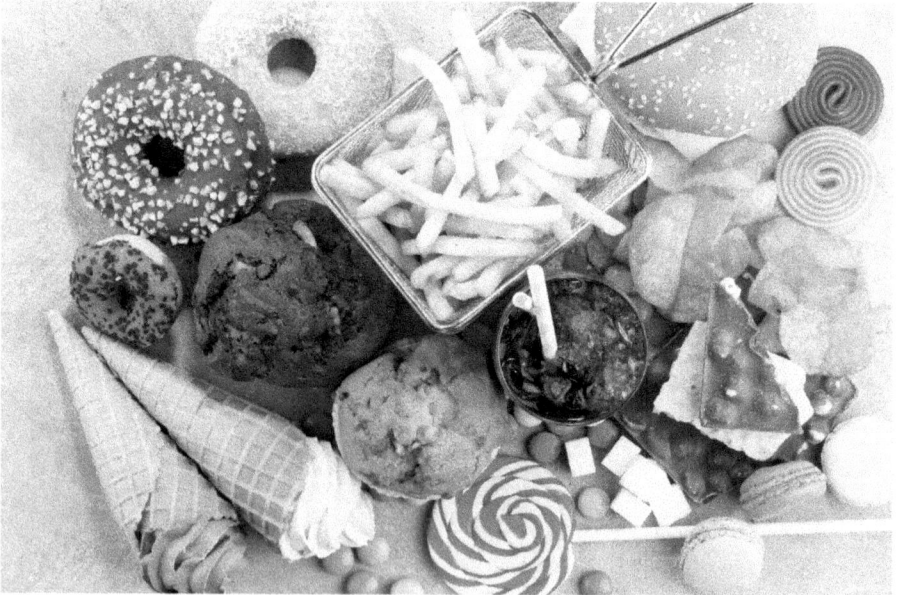

For you were bought at a price; therefore glorify God in your body and in your spirit, which are God's. 1 Corinthians 6:20

I n this section, I'm going to give you a list of foods that you should eliminate from your diet for different reasons, but since we were on the subject of the small intestine, let's begin here. I will probably break your heart, but here goes.

GLUTEN

What if I told you that the bowl of oatmeal you are so fond of having each morning could threaten your immunity and resistance to invaders such as COVID-19? Does this seem far-fetched to you? Let me explain. Wheat, rye, barley, and oats all contain a sticky protein called gluten that, after many years of consumption, destroys essential tissue in the small intestine and lessens immunity. These tiny raised finger-shaped tissues are called villi, and their job is to absorb calories and nutrients from foods. This sticky gluten, or in the case of oats, gliadin, a component of gluten, adheres to the lining of the small intestine. The word gluten comes from the word "glue," not by coincidence. After a considerable accumulation of this sticky protein develops in the small intestine, gluten intolerance, a common occurrence, takes place with a majority of people. Gluten intolerance can go on unnoticed but is still causing harm to the digestive system. After many years of consumption, the tiny villi no longer function. Those vitamins and minerals you have been taking for health benefits will pass through bodily functions with little or no absorption ever taking place. The old saying, "You are what you eat" doesn't hold. The truth is that you are what you absorb.

It is unknown why the digestion of gluten is so hard for the stomach to digest. Maybe because wheat is grass and although man discovered a way to process the seed of this grass, it remains a food meant for ruminants. What is a ruminant? True ruminants, such as cattle, sheep, goats, deer, and antelope, have one stomach with four compartments: the rumen, reticulum, omasum, and abomasums. The ruminant stomach occupies almost 75 percent of the abdominal cavity, filling nearly all of the left side and extending significantly into the right side. The relative size of the four compartments is as follows: the rumen and reticulum comprise 84 percent of the volume of the total stomach, the omasum 12 percent, and the abomasum 4 percent. The rumen is the largest stomach compartment, holding up to 40 gallons in a mature cow. The short of it is, It takes a stomach with four compartments for a ruminant to digest grass, and you only have one.

Bread has always been "The Staff of Life," so how could this ever have been? It seems illogical according to history. Consider this. In ancient times man did not have use of the technology that exists today, and wheat has been severely tampered with through hybridization and genetic modification to become resistant to glyphosate (Roundup).

ROUNDUP (GLYPHOSATE)

Recently a lawsuit was filed against The Monsanto Company (now owned by Bayer) by a farmer and his wife, who both claimed that Monsanto failed to warn of the cancer risks in using its Roundup product. The discovery in that lawsuit led to the following conclusions stated in Gammon (2009) below:

Until now, most health studies have focused on the safety of glyphosate, rather than the mixture of ingredients found in Roundup. But in the new study, scientists found that Roundup's inert ingredients amplified the toxic effect on human cells—even at concentrations much more diluted than those used on farms and lawns.

One specific inert ingredient, polyethoxylated tallow amine, or POEA, was more deadly to human embryonic, placental and umbilical cord cells than the herbicide itself – a finding the researchers call 'astonishing.'

'This clearly confirms that the [inert ingredients] in Roundup formulations are not inert,' wrote the study authors from France's University of Caen. 'Moreover, the proprietary mixtures available on the market could cause cell damage and even death [at the] residual levels' found on Roundup-treated crops, such as soybeans, alfalfa, and corn, or lawns and gardens.'[1]

Simply put, the wheat of today is not the wheat of Biblical times. The mere fact that it and the mineral-deficient ground it grows in, drenched in toxic chemicals, should be enough reason to stay away. But I digress. Let's get back to the part where I break your heart by the elimination of these products and their derivatives from your diet.

- Bread/Pastries
- Pasta
- Cookies/Cakes
- Crackers
- Pie Crust
- Bagels
- Oatmeal
- Granola
- Beer
- Soy sauce
- White vinegar
- Tomato soup
- Sausage
- Scrambled eggs (i.e., pre-packaged)

The above-bulleted list is only a partial list as wheat hides in so many processed foods when used as a thickener (gluten). You have to read the labels on everything. Even if products like oatmeal or cereals like Cheerios say "gluten-free," be aware that they contain gliadin, which is a component of gluten that produces the same result.

For those who cannot do without having baked bread, there are always gluten-free alternatives. But their consumption should be approached with caution because they all raise blood sugar levels just as quickly as wheat. Usually, these processed foods contain almond flour, brown or white rice flour, tapioca flour, potato starch, or a combination of thereof. Too many carbohydrates still cause sugar spikes and elevated blood sugar levels, which may lead to pre-diabetes, type II diabetes, and many other accompanying ailments if the consumption is not limited.

OILS IN A BOTTLE

Some oils include great benefits for the human body, namely omega-3 and omega 9. These are both essential fatty acids (EFAs) because they are vital to our health and must be obtained from food sources as our cells cannot make them. On the other hand, omega 6 is always in abundance and readily consumed in an oxidized form. Without the accompanying 3 and 9 factors, omega-6 alone demonstrates a burden to the body because it causes inflammation and contributes to various chronic ailments. Atherosclerosis, heart disease, diabetes, obesity, uterine fibroids, endometriosis, arthritis, and more result from a lack of omega 3 and 9.

The three enemies of oil are air, heat, and light. What makes these the enemy of oil? They all cause oxidation of the oil. Oxidized oil isn't fit for human consumption. It is systematically dousing yourself with free radicals. You take vitamins and minerals to eliminate free radicals yet; for example, every time that you eat a french fry, you add plenty of free radicals to your system.

The absolute worst you can do to your body comes from the consumption of fried foods. When heating any kind of oil, the chemical structure of it changes. Heating oils create dreaded trans-fats, acrylamides, and heterocyclic amines. These types of free radicals lead to cancer.

Heat, used in deodorizing, hydrogenation (to make margarines and shortenings), and commercial frying and deep-frying used to make consumer items, destroys EFAs by twisting their molecules from a natural *cis*-shape to an unnatural *trans*-shape.[2]

While It is common to find olive oil in bottles manufactured with dark glass to protect its content from the element of light, the problems with heat and Oxygen still have not been addressed. I believe that the reason for this is mainly to preserve olive oil's unique taste.

> **Light**, the greatest enemy of EFAs produces free radicals in oils and speeds up the reaction of oils with Oxygen from the air by 1000 times, resulting in rancid oil. . . Light destroys the vital biological properties of the EFAs.[3]

We find EFAs in fatty fish, krill, flax seeds, hemp seeds, borage roots, and evening primrose roots. But when packaged in a bottle, they will oxidize with time. Yes, although stored in a refrigerated form, where the light and heat problem may be solved, EFAs in a bottle still have air trapped inside the container. As the product diminishes, more air is trapped inside, causing increased oxidation.

> **Oxygen**, even in the absence of light, breaks down EFAs. The result is what we know as rancid oil, which has a scratchy, bitter, fishy, or painty taste, r a characteristic unpleasant smell, like a parking lot in August heat. Dozens of breakdown produces form, with toxic or unknown effects on our body's functions.[4]

FRIED FOOD

As stated above, heat is one of the biggest enemies of oil because it alters the chemistry of the oil. One of the by-products of heating oil is trans-fat. Trans fat not only adds to your LDL cholesterol levels, but it also decreases your HDL cholesterol. HDL cholesterol mistakenly referred to as "good cholesterol" and LDL as "bad cholesterol" is essential to be kept in balance. Stated incorrectly, what needs to be understood is that both types of cholesterol are harmful once oxidation takes place. However, for the sake of this discussion, what happens when eating fried and deep-fried foods is the consumption of nothing but oxidized oil, which brings more oxidative stress to the body.

HOW TRANS FAT HARMS YOU

Below is the opinion of The Mayo Clinic on trans fats.

Doctors worry about added trans fat because it increases the risk for heart attacks, stroke and type 2 diabetes. Trans fat also has an unhealthy effect on your cholesterol levels. . . If the fatty deposits within your arteries tear or rupture, a blood clot may form and block blood flow to a part of your heart, causing a heart attack; or to a part of your brain, causing a stroke.[5]

Lately, consumer awareness has risen, involving hydrogenated fats in foods due to plentiful media exposure. Manufacturers now have labels on their products that they hope will gain the public confidence and steer the public to their brand over the competition's brand. Now that the public knows these fats cannot assimilate effectively after ingestion and can cling to the arteries contributing to atherosclerosis or hardening of the arteries, they are bad news. Nevertheless, did you know that creating hydrogenated oils has the potential to introduce heavy metals such as aluminum and nickel into the body? In the book "Fats That Heal Fats That Kill" the author states,

---

Margarines and shortenings contribute the bulk of the trans-fatty acids found in the human diet. We consume about 40 grams of margarines daily, and they average 20% or more trans-fatty acids. The effects of these altered fatty acids on our body moved the Dutch government to ban the sale of margarines containing trans-fatty acids.[6]

Fried foods are so bad for you that people working in restaurants who breathe in the fumes from heated oils are more susceptible to developing lung cancer and other cancers. The National Institutes of Health in 2017 said,

> The animal products served at fast food restaurants are making the health of the population much worse, creating dangerous carcinogens from the food being grilled, barbecued, and fried at high temperatures. The World Health Organization has classified processed meats (hot dogs, sausage, bacon, and lunch meats) a class 1 carcinogen. AGEs are also highest in barbecued and fried animal products which also contain cancer-causing chemicals such as heterocyclic amines, polycyclic aromatic hydrocarbons, and lipid peroxidases, which are mutagenic.[7]

In 2015, Gadiraju made the connection between trans fat and hypertension:

> The process of oxidation during frying food increases the amount of trans-fatty acids in food and is positively associated with the risk of hypertension.[8]

Trans fat leads to hypertension, and hypertension can lead to the production of small tears in the arteries. Cholesterol gets the job of repairing these tears in the arterial walls and, over time, will cause the narrowing of that artery where the tears once existed. The cholesterol is just doing its natural job, so having much cholesterol is not of too much concern because it makes up 70% of the brain and 90% of all hormones. More important is whether the cholesterol is becoming oxidized through the diet and any other contributing factors to the individual's habits.

BURNT ANIMAL FAT

Many MDs have given the consumption of fats a negative connotation because they have not received enough education about nutrition. According to a 2015 report in the Journal of Biomedical Education, only 29 percent of US medical schools offer the recommended 25 hours of nutrition education to med students. This report further concludes,

It cannot be a realistic expectation for physicians to effectively address obesity, diabetes, metabolic syndrome, hospital malnutrition, and many other conditions as long as they are not taught during medical school and residency training how to recognize and treat the nutritional root causes.[9]

According to a 2010 report in Academic Medicine, US medical schools offer only 19.6 hours of nutrition education on average, across four years of medical school. Armed with these factors, why would anyone want to consult with an MD about preventing chronic disease or prevention by dietary measures when the MDs goal is just to treat the particular ailment and bill the insurance company repeatedly?

OK, so now that we know who not to listen to, listen to this. Burnt animal fats are a problem for the human body. The reason being that well-done meats are not only more challenging to digest, but the charring of the flesh at high temperatures creates a carcinogenic chemical substance. That substance is Heterocyclic Amines (HCAs). When the amino acids and proteins present in muscle meats react to very high temperatures in cooking, forming HCAs. Another substance formed during grilling, baking, frying, or roasting is acrylamide, a cancer-causing agent.

BAKED POTATO SKINS

As you are probably aware, the Russet potato's skin is known to contain the most nutrition as opposed to the inside. However, as with the cooking and preparation of meat, this depends upon how the preparation of the potato. The only way to consider eating the skin of any potato is by boiling it. When a potato boils, it only reaches a temperature of no more than 212 degrees. This temperature will prevent the formation of acrylamide.

In comparison, roasting a potato usually requires a temperature of 400 degrees and above. Acrylamide appears at high levels in foods that become browned during the cooking process. A tell-tale sign is grill marks. Yet foods such as french fries, potato chips, pretzels, cereals, grilled vegetables, and dried fruits also contain acrylamide. That said, the primary culprit for acrylamide is cigarette smoke. Smokers get the double-whammy from inhaling burning tobacco, and if you live with a smoker, you do too.

If you are serious about your health like me, you will discover that dining out is difficult because of the way food preparation takes place. Cooking at home is always the healthiest solution because it is there that you can control how you prepare your food. The next time you visit a restaurant that makes appetizers for consumption as you wait upon your meal, count how many of these delights are FRIED or GRILLED. Although this may be the quickest way to satisfy your hunger and craving for food, it is not the best way. Think twice before ordering an appetizer-especially those roasted potato skins with sour cream, cheese, and bacon!

PROCESSED MEATS

Any meats containing nitrates or nitrites are processed meats. Nitrates used to preserve meats give them a longer shelf life. Some examples of processed meats are pepperoni, corned beef, Spam, salami, bologna, hot dogs, bacon, jerky, sausage, and more. It matters not whether the source of sodium nitrate is chemical or from celery juice (a natural source of nitrate). When nitrates convert to nitrite, it is toxic to the body. Nitrites in processed meats are close to proteins (specifically amino acids). When cooked at high temperatures, a cancer-causing compound called nitrosamines are easily formed.

The conversion to nitrite and further metabolism of nitrogen compounds to nitrosamines is related to negative effects of nitrate to consumers since is associated with the risk of gastrointestinal cancer.[10]

When it comes down to the consumption of these meats, I need to convince you to "JUST SAY NO." Processed meats are known to contain carcinogens that heating only amplifies.

Nitrates can react with amino acids to form nitrosamines, which have been reported to cause cancer in animals [Bruning-Fann and Kaneene 1993]. Elevated risk of non-Hodgkin's lymphoma [Ward et al. 1996] and cancers of the esophagus, nasopharynx, bladder, colon, prostate and thyroid have been reported [Cantor 1997; Eichholzer and Gutzwiller 1998; Barrett et al. 1998; Ward et al. 2010].[11]

CARBONATED BEVERAGES WITH A MEAL

Soda, pop, beer (which is like liquid bread), fizzy wine coolers, or carbonated water are better as stand-alone beverages and not for consumption with a meal. For proper digestion to take place, stomach acid should have a low Ph level, usually of about 1.0. Most people have low stomach acid due to a couple of reasons. First, the lack of calcium which the body uses to squirt the acid into the stomach as calcium is lacking from the diet, and secondly, because medical doctors are erroneously cautioning people to use less salt to avoid hypertension. Drinking a carbonated beverage anywhere from one hour before a meal, during a meal, or to within the hour after completion of a meal can affect the digestive process negatively by raising the Ph level of the stomach even more.

It is our recommendation in addition to making sure that your calcium intake is adequate, always to salt your food to taste. However, the quality of the salt is essential. Salt that is pure white (like common table salt) is void of trace minerals. Some of these salt products are made from petroleum, while others are sea salt, but the bleaching process removes all the trace minerals. Sometimes these manufactured salts also contain sugar.

These table salts being void of trace minerals lead to swelling, liver problems, hypertension, heart disease, muscle cramps, stroke, heart failure, edema, water retention, PMS, anxiety, and nervous system disorders when consumed in excess. The body requires more water to flush the mineral-deficient salt out of the system. Himalayan, Celtic, and Russian salts vary in color, but the one thing they have in common is that they still contain the healthy trace minerals. This salt is needed by the body to produce hydrochloric acid, which aids in digestion because sodium chloride is a component of hydrochloric acid.

---

1. Gammon, C. (2009) Weed-Whacking Herbicide Proves Deadly to Human Cells. Environmental Health News [Scientificamerican.com]
2. Erasmus, U. (1986) Caring For Essential Fatty Acids. In *Fats That Heal Fats That Kill*. (2nd ed.) Burnaby BC Canada; Alive Books. pp. 53-54
3. Erasmus, U. (1986) Caring For Essential Fatty Acids. In *Fats That Heal Fats That Kill*. (2nd ed.) Burnaby BC Canada; Alive Books. pp. 53-54
4. Erasmus, U. (1986) Caring For Essential Fatty Acids. In *Fats That Heal Fats That Kill*. (2nd ed.) Burnaby BC Canada; Alive Books. pp. 53-54
5. MFMER (2020). Trans Fat Is Double Trouble For Your Heart Health. [Mayoclinic.org]
6. Erasmus, U. (1986) From Oil To Margarine. In Fats That Heal Fats That Kill. (2nd ed.) Burnaby BC Canada; Alive Books. P. 104
7. Furhman, J. (2017). The Hidden Dangers Of Fast And Processed Food. [PMC free article]
8. Gadiraju, T. V., Patel, Y., Gaziano, J. M., & Djoussé, L. (2015). Fried Food Consumption and Cardiovascular Health: A Review of Current Evidence. Nutrients, 7(10), 8424–8430. https://doi.org/10.3390/nu7105404
9. Adams, K., et al., (2015) The State of Nutrition Education at US Medical Schools. Hindawi Publishing Corporation, Journal of Biomedical Education, Volume 2015, Article ID 357627 P. 1 https://www.hindawi.com/journals/jbe/2015/357627/
10. Karwowska, M., & Kononiuk, A. (2020). Nitrates/Nitrites in Food-Risk for Nitrosative Stress and Benefits. Antioxidants (Basel, Switzerland), 9(3), 241. https://doi.org/10.3390/antiox9030241
11. What Are the Health Effects from Exposure to Nitrates and Nitrites? (2020) US Department of Health and Human Services, Agency for Toxic Substances and Disease Registry p. 56 https://www.atsdr.cdc.gov/csem/csem.asp?csem=28&po=10

Chapter Four

STEP 3: EAT HEALTHILY

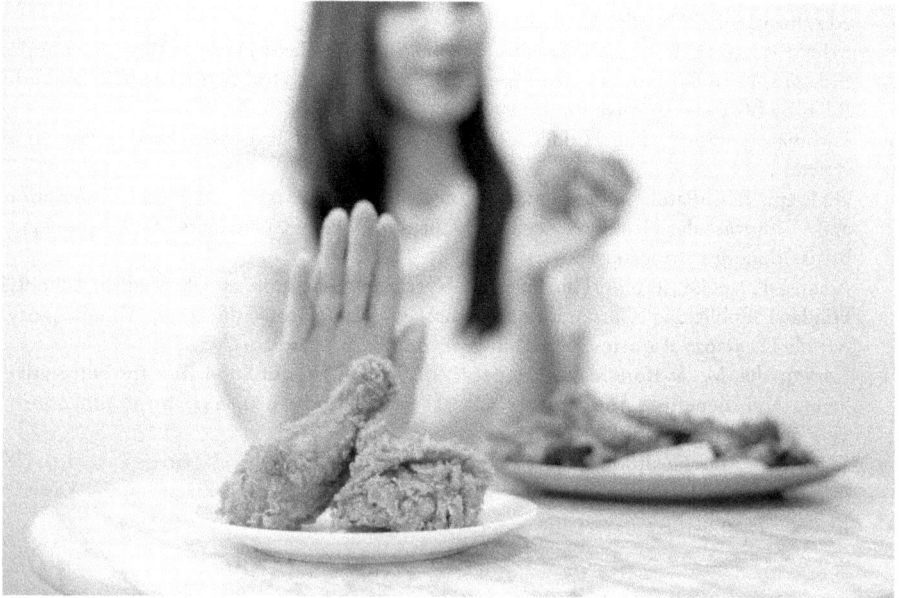

Beloved, I pray that you may prosper in all things and be in health, just as your soul prospers. 3 John 2

So now that I've covered for you what not to eat, you're probably asking what's left that's good to eat? Here's a partial list:
- Eggs—soft scrambled in butter, soft boiled, or poached.
- Salt
- Butter/Lard
- Dairy
- Fish
- Chicken
- Pork
- Lamb
- Beef—rare/medium rare only, grass-fed is preferred
- Veggies
- Fruit
- Mixed, Salted Nuts—no peanuts
- Nut Butters—no extra sugar
- Rice
- Millet
- Pure Buckwheat (Isn't wheat)
- Beans
- Couscous (made from pearl millet only)
- Quinoa
- Corn – as long as it is non-GMO
- Coffee, Tea, Green tea, Red wine
- 4-8, 8 oz glasses of filtered water each day. Avoid soft plastic bottles.

See, there are still many other food choices, but now you have been cautioned as to what ways to avoid preparing some of them to improve your health.

If you are someone who has made a choice not to consume any meat, let me warn you that supplementation is even more critical, mainly if you work out. As the average American consumes about 100 grams of protein a day, being plant-based may require that you include even more food into your diet. While it is possible to derive amounts of necessary proteins from plants, carbohydrate consumption will also go up as will the number of calories. Vegetarians who do not supplement make some of the unhealthiest people on the planet. Meat protein is more concentrated than vegetables, and therefore the derived benefits come by less consumption. Green, leafy vegetables are about 50% protein, so spinach, kale, and collard greens are beneficial. About 10 to 15 grams of protein come from either a cup of beans, peas, or lentils, but two slices of whole-grain bread will only provide about 10 grams of protein and also cause a rapid rise in blood sugar because grains convert to glucose very quickly.

I am not on a mission to convince anyone that they should eat meat, and there are plentiful reasons to avoid particular meats, poultry, and fish. My emphasis is on supplementation, whether you are a carnivore or not, because the nutrition is lacking in whatever you decide to eat, whether plant-based or not.

CARNIVOROUS CONSIDERATIONS

The nutrition derived from animal protein stems from what that animal ate in its diet. Unfortunately, farm-raised seafood is tremendously deficient in food value, and mercury levels are incredibly high in certain species. Wild-caught seafood is more expensive in stores than farm-raised for a reason. For example, the packaging of farm-raised salmon includes typically the words "color added" because next to wild-caught salmon, without added coloring, it would appear grey in color. The grey, unappetizing color would turn off most seafood lovers, hence the added color. The wild salmon is not confined to nets in the ocean, allowing them to partake in their natural diet, high in astaxanthin, a reddish pigment that belongs to a group of chemicals called carotenoids that comes from certain algae. These algae are what give pink flamingos their color as well as shrimp, lobster, trout, and other seafood.

Below, in Menon (2016), we are cautioned about seafood to avoid.

Avoid a few key species. King mackerel, marlin, orange roughy, shark, swordfish, tilefish, ahi tuna, and bigeye tuna all contain high levels of mercury. Women who are pregnant or nursing or who plan to become pregnant within a year should avoid eating these fish. So should children younger than six.

Ease up on tuna. Tuna is the most common source of mercury

exposure in the country. If you or your kids regularly eat canned tuna, stick to light or skipjack tuna, and limit it to less than two servings a week. A 130-pound woman can eat almost two six-ounce cans of light tuna a week and stay within the EPA-recommended safe zone for mercury. A four- or five-year-old child should eat only about four ounces of light tuna per week. The rules change when it comes to albacore tuna. Children should avoid that fish altogether, and women of childbearing age should stick to no more than four ounces per week.[1]

The animal's diet harbors the same considerations as with any farm-raised animal. Animals raised in close confinement tend not to be as healthy as those the one that roams. Only recently has poultry been given more time to mature without the aid of additional hormones to accelerate growth. When these chickens that lived their entire lives in cages with no ability to exercise, they grew with huge breasts but often had not enough musculature to walk and carry their weight. The benefits were to farmers' pocketbooks because, in a shorter amount of time, they would produce the favorite meat of many Americans, chicken breast. As it was, many chickens would die before being slaughtered because their undeveloped hearts couldn't take the strain of supporting their immense bodies.

Another factor to consider is the use of toxic chemicals on the production of the animal's feed. The farming industry feeds a laboratory constructed diet to keep an animal alive long enough for slaughter at the lowest possible cost to maximize profits. For this reason, the American government has chosen to subsidize farmers to produce large amounts of corn. Besides producing valuable ethanol from corn for use as a gasoline additive, the farmers feed this glyphosate-laced (Roundup) corn to all farm-raised animals.

Farmers give a lifetime diet of GMO crops to pigs, chickens, and cows that have been sprayed season after season with glyphosate. The limits on the amount of glyphosate allowed in animal feed are much higher than it is for people. Vicini says:

The weight of the evidence suggests that glyphosate use in crops fed to poultry and livestock has not affected animal health, rumen/gut microbes or production without affecting the safety of consuming meat, milk, and eggs.[2]

1. Menon, S. (2016). Mercury Guide. Natural Resources Defense Council https://www.nrdc.org/stories/mercury-guide#:~:text=King%20mackerel%2C%20marlin%2C%20orange%20roughy,should%20avoid%20eating%20these%20fish.
2. Vicini, J. L., Reeves, W. R., Swarthout, J. T., & Karberg, K. A. (2019). Glyphosate in livestock: feed residues and animal health1. Journal of animal science, 97(11), 4509–4518. https://doi.org/10.1093/jas/skz295

Chapter Five

STEP 4: MANAGE STRESS LEVELS

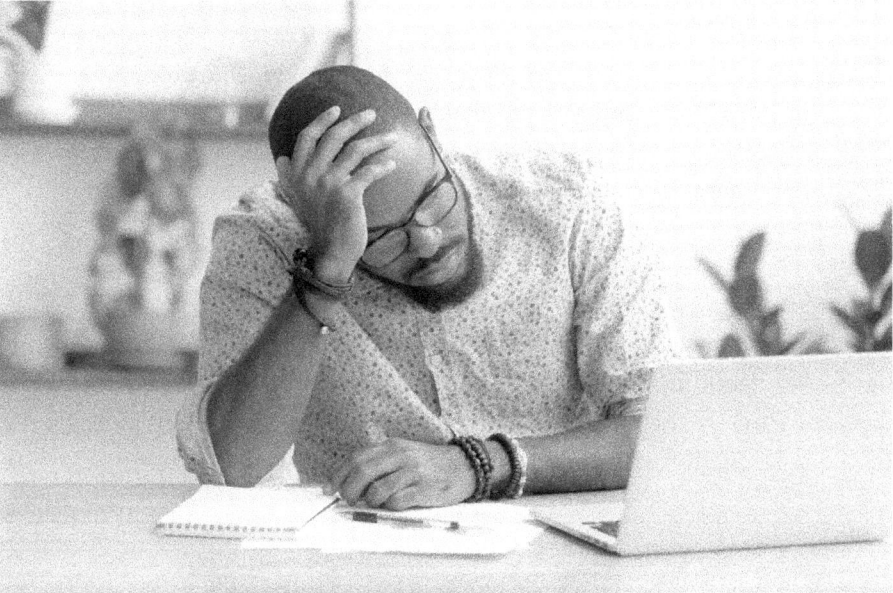

For to be carnally minded is death, but to be spiritually minded is life and peace. Romans 8:6

One of the most important things you can do to boost your immune system's capabilities is to manage your stress levels. Stress affects the nervous system, which consists of two parts, 1) The sympathetic nervous system (SNS), which channels our energy into the things that keep us alive in emergency and life-threatening situations, and 2) the parasympathetic system (PNS) which takes over during more long-term activities. The PNS is the place in which we want our nervous systems to abide rather than the SNS, commonly known as "fight or flight" mode. When our nervous systems remain in the PNS mode, it adds to our longevity because this so-called "rest and digest" mode adds to our health and well-being.

In Morey, we find the best reason why the fight or flight hormone, cortisol, is best kept under control as much as possible.

Cortisol is ordinarily anti-inflammatory and contains the immune response, but chronic elevations can lead to the immune system becoming "resistant," an accumulation of stress hormones, and increased production of inflammatory cytokines that further compromise the immune response.[1]

Stress And COVID-19

It is important to note that some people experience a "cytokine storm" during an encounter with the latest coronavirus called COVID-19. The danger of this is that the storm is an overreaction to the threat triggered by the host nervous system. In COVID-19 Basics, we learn that:

When this happens, the immune system attacks the body's own tissues, potentially causing significant harm. A cytokine storm triggers an exaggerated inflammatory response that may damage the liver, blood vessels, kidneys, and lungs, and increase formation of blood clots throughout the body. Ultimately, the cytokine storm may cause more harm than the coronavirus itself.[2]

We know that Vitamin D is responsible for regulating the immune system and the production of these cytokines. Therefore, a deficiency in this vitamin leads to an overall immune system deficiency. Vitamin D is produced by sunlight through absorption by the skin; however, those with more melanin in their skin tend to absorb less, so the conversion may or may not take place depending on the length of exposure. Consequently, people with darker skin, as well as people who populate those areas that have limited sunlight during the year, definitely should supplement with Vitamin D.

We now know that COVID-19 is a respiratory ailment that, with progression, can adversely affect the proper functioning of other significant organs in the body that may lead to death. In Assimakopoulos, we read:

> Accumulating evidence suggests that a subgroup of patients with severe COVID-19 might have a cytokine storm syndrome associated with acute respiratory distress syndrome (ARDS), multiple organ failure, and increased mortality.[3]

It is important to note that fear of COVID-19 and not being able to receive enough Oxygen through normal breathing are in opposition to each other. In this case, fear is the enemy and the biggest liar. Being diagnosed with COVID-19 doesn't mean that you will die from it, but it does mean that it is essential to control stress levels to facilitate normal breathing. As the heart rate increases, so does the need for extra Oxygen, and the lungs may now be experiencing diminished capacity. In this situation, relaxation, although difficult, is of the utmost importance to calm the nervous system and avoid a possible cytokine storm from the body's unregulated negative response.

SUPPLEMENTATION THAT MAY HELP FIGHT CYTOKINE STORM

We are now aware of the importance of Vitamin D in regulating the body's immune system by the autopsies performed on those who have succumbed to the disease. Also discussed in Assimakopoulos 2020, are the benefits of supplementation with N-Acetyl L-Cysteine (NAC) in patients with COVID-19:

> The results of these studies offer reasonable basis for the addition of 1200 mg/d oral NAC on therapeutic schemes of patients with COVID-19, as a measure that could potentially prevent the development of the cytokine storm syndrome and ARDS.[4]

NAC, as well as the mineral selenium, are known to be precursors for the production of glutathione. Further, in Horowitz 2020, we discover that:

> Two patients living in New York City (NYC) with a history of Lyme and tick-borne co-infections experienced a cough and dyspnea and demonstrated radiological findings consistent with novel coronavirus pneumonia (NCP). A trial of 2 g of PO or IV glutathione was used in both patients and improved their dyspnea within 1 h of use. Repeated use of both 2000 mg of PO and IV glutathione was effective in further relieving respiratory symptoms.
>
> Conclusion: Oral and IV glutathione, glutathione precursors (N-acetyl-cysteine) and alpha lipoic acid may represent a novel treatment approach for blocking NFKappaB and addressing 'cytokine storm syndrome' and respiratory distress in patients with COVID-19 pneumonia.[5]

In extreme cases of a patient not being able to control this aspect of respiration while coupled with fear, MDs consider using a ventilator.

However, a person's body needs to breathe on its own rather than mechanically as it aids the body's natural healing defenses. I understand a physician's desire to save a life, but in many cases, a ventilator may cause irreparable harm and cause the patient to expire.

In these uncertain times, many things happen outside of our control. It is essential to do the best and be the best person that you can and thereby strengthen the things you can control. In short, work on yourself. Do everything possible to eliminate the stress you are aware of in your life, but don't overburden your digestive system by adding only the foods that provide you with comfort. Eating the wrong foods will add stress to your body without you even knowing it until afterward.

---

1. Morey, J. N., Boggero, I. A., Scott, A. B., & Segerstrom, S. C. (2015). Current Directions in Stress and Human Immune Function. Current opinion in psychology, 5, 13–17. https://doi.org/10.1016/j.copsyc.2015.03.007

2. COVID-19 basics - Symptoms, spread and other essential information about the new coronavirus and COVID-19. (2020) Harvard Health Publishing https://www.health.harvard.edu/diseases-and-conditions/covid-19-basics

3. Assimakopoulos, S. F., & Marangos, M. (2020). N-acetyl-cysteine may prevent COVID-19-associated cytokine storm and acute respiratory distress syndrome. Medical hypotheses, 140, 109778. Advance online publication. https://doi.org/10.1016/j.mehy.2020.109778

4. Assimakopoulos, S. F., & Marangos, M. (2020). N-acetyl-cysteine may prevent COVID-19-associated cytokine storm and acute respiratory distress syndrome. Medical hypotheses, 140, 109778. Advance online publication. https://doi.org/10.1016/j.mehy.2020.109778

5. Horowitz, Richard I et al. Efficacy of glutathione therapy in relieving dyspnea associated with COVID-19 pneumonia: A report of 2 cases. Respiratory medicine case reports, vol. 30 101063. April 21. 2020, doi:10.1016/j.rmcr.2020.101063

Chapter Six

STEP 5: EXERCISE AND SLEEP

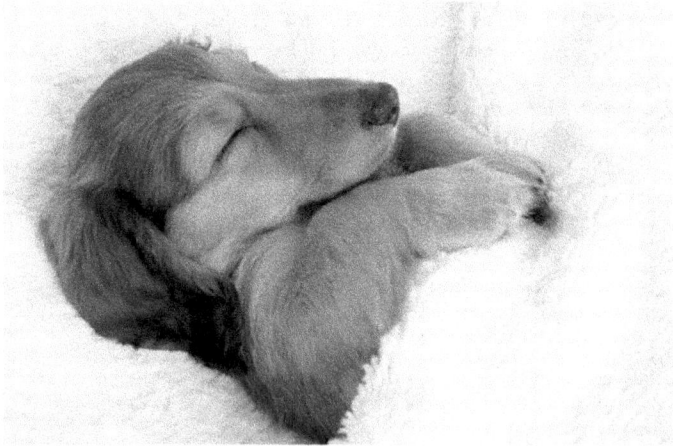

For bodily exercise profits a little, but godliness is profitable for all things, having promise of the life that now is and of that which is to come. 1 Timothy 4:8 NKJV

EXERCISE

A saying that speaks volumes to me is one that says, "Fitness is 20% exercise and 80% nutrition. You can't outrun your fork." After understanding both the preceding statement and 1 Timothy 4:8, I conclude that although exercise is essential, nutrition is even more critical. But first, let's discuss the activity.

Many young people would like to have an outstanding physique to be admired by the opposite sex. They will spend many hours in a gym working on specific muscles to enhance their image of themselves. Others are athletes who want to strength train for endurance on the playing field when in competition. As one progressively ages, the thought of this type of training may prompt them to visit the refrigerator, then the television remote on their way to the couch. Whatever your frame of mind, you will need to exercise. The warning that I give is to be sure that before exerting yourself, you have nutrified yourself properly—not having that 80% of nutrition can prove to be suicidal.

We have heard of young, healthy athletes suddenly dropping dead on the field. Reggie Lewis, 27, who played for the Boston Celtics, collapsed while shooting baskets at the team's training center. A 22-year old graduate of the University of Colorado, Darren Mallot, collapsed and died on the basketball court in Boulder, Colorado following a lay-up. A 17-year old junior in North Bergen, N.J., Jackson Muamba, collapsed and later died during a basketball game. All these athletes known to be specimens of health died from some sort of heart failure. I'll add this just to reinforce the point. Dr. Gail L. Clark, a Cardiologist and Head of the cardiac reha-bilitation program at St. Luke's Hospital in west St. Louis County, died after suffering a heart attack at age 47. Dr. Robert Paine, a cardiologist and clinical professor at Washington University School of Medicine, is quoted in The St. Louis Post-Dispatch as saying, "She was highly respected as a cardiologist and a leader in the field of stress medicine as it relates to heart disease." (Wallach, J. 1994) She left behind a husband, two daughters, two sons, her mother, two sisters, and two brothers. Let's hope they are not following her advice alone.

Why did these people die so young? The answer lies in the lack of nutrition. Your body requires it, but it does not get it solely from the intake of non-nutritious foods from depleted soils. You have read that plants and various meats contain vitamins, and that is true. However, plants and animals do not create minerals; they come from the ground. But they only come from the ground if the land contains them. The cow's milk and by-products that you believe in providing calcium most likely do not contain as much calcium as maple syrup. Minerals are the catalysts that cause vitamins to go into action. Without minerals, vitamins are barely helpful.

When an athlete or, for that matter, anyone sweats, the sweat is not just water. The sweat is a soup that contains minerals that your body was holding. Sweat tastes salty because you have consumed sodium chloride, a salty tasting mineral beneficial for things like digestion and, oh yes, electrolytes that produce electricity that keeps your heart beating. If you have been sweating and your body doesn't have an abundance of minerals, you put yourself at risk, and the suicide aspect enters. Call it accidental suicide.

I'm not trying to put fear into your hearts, but I am trying to tell you how important maintaining the 80% nutrition is to your well-being. Meanwhile, here is a list of the benefits you can achieve just from walking for 30 minutes a day.

- Reduces the risk of heart disease
- Helps to maintain your weight
- Reduces your stress levels
- Increases your energy levels
- Helps to boost your mood
- Increases blood circulation
- Prevents obesity
- Can help to reduce anxiety
- Increases functioning of the lungs
- Increases the body's access to Vitamin D
- Reduces the risk of cancer
- Can improve the quality of sleep
- Gives you time to practice self-care
- Improves coordination and balance
- Improves quality of life
- Reduces the chance of diabetes

- Walking can spark creativity
- Strengthens bones and muscles
- Can improve blood pressure
- Can help boost your immune system

SLEEP

Calcium is the most prevalent mineral in the body and stored in the bones. Many people think that once the bones form and a person reaches their height—that's it, and no more growth takes place. They are wrong because your bones are working for you all the time. That means that they also need rest, and when you sleep, that is when any calcium that you received during the day, whether from food or supplementation, is absorbed back into them.

The benefits of sleep are numerous, with the main one being the filtering of your blood by your liver. According to Chinese medicine, 1-3 a.m. is the time the body should be asleep because toxins released from the body begins the production of fresh new blood. Porter (2017) gives us a list of some of the other benefits.

- Better physical health. Sleep boosts your immune system, and you will likely get sick less often. Plus, you will likely have more energy throughout the day.
- Reduces the risk for serious medical conditions such as type 2 diabetes, high blood pressure, and heart disease
- Helps maintain healthy body weight. Sleep is a vital player in your body's ability to regulate hormones that control your appetite and metabolism. Many of us crave carbohydrates when we are tired.
- Lowers stress and improves your mood
- Helps you focus and think more creatively. Sleep may ease your ability to solve problems and remember important information.
- Improves relationships. You may find that you are more patient when you have slept well.
- Reduces injuries. When it comes to driving, sleep deprivation is like being intoxicated; sleepy drivers cause thousands of car

accidents every year. Well-rested people are more alert, make better decisions, and use better judgment.[1]

To sum it all up, sleep provides the best time for the physical restoration of all the body's organs. You can't eat while sleeping, so the body goes into a fasting mode facilitating healing. According to the Traditional Chinese Organ Body Clock, 9-11 p.m. is when one should be sleeping so the body can conserve energy for the following day. 11 p.m. to 1 a.m. is the time of the Gall Bladder, and the body should be at rest to feel energized upon waking. 1-3 a.m. is the time of the liver when the toxins accumulated from the day are released, and new blood replenished. 3-5 a.m. is the time of the lungs, and when restocking the body with Oxygen, the body should be kept warm. If awake at this time, one may benefit by breathing exercises, or by drinking hot peppermint tea.

---

1. Porter, Lucinda K. (2017) Sleep: the Key to a Healthy Liver. Retrieved August 7, 2020, from http://www.hepmag.com/article/sleep-key-healthy-liver

Chapter Seven

STEP 6: SUPPLEMENT WITH MEDICAL NUTRITION

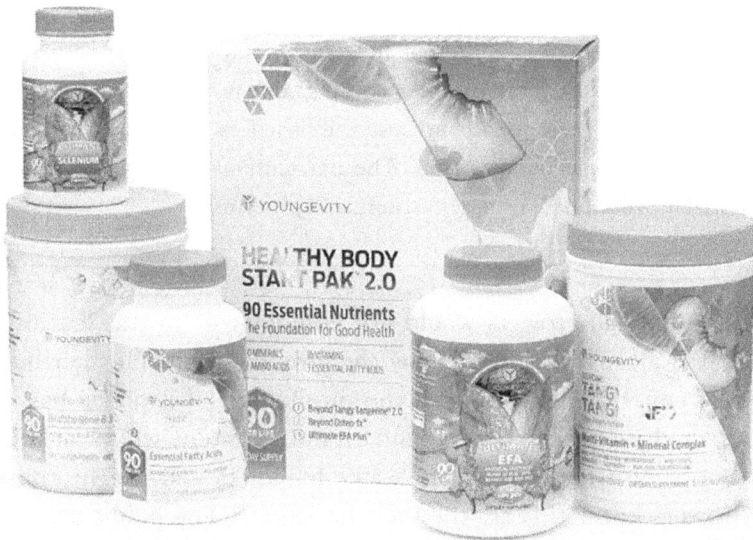

Youngevity Healthy Body Brain and Heart Pak

"And God said, "See, I have given you every herb that yields seed which is on the face of all the earth, and every tree whose fruit yields seed; to you it shall be for food." Genesis 1:29

LACK OF NUTRITION IN FOODS

Commercial farming does not take into consideration Scripture found in Leviticus 25:4, which reads, "But in the seventh year the land is to have a year of sabbath rest, a sabbath to the Lord. Do not sow your fields or prune your vineyards." This Scripture makes it clear the land is supposed to rest. Allowing this process to take place is a way for exhausted soil to be restored with the elements necessary for our nutrition when growing our food.

Commercially grown fruits and vegetables have proven to show diminished levels of six different nutrients when compared with the nutrient levels of the 1950s according to new findings by the University of Texas researchers and published in the Journal of the American College of Nutrition. The nutrients affected are calcium, riboflavin, vitamin C, iron, potassium, and protein.[1]

The commercial growers would not comment as to this loss of nutrition, but it is all revealed in the way the growers approach their business. The use of genetic engineering in the production of produce has significantly affected its nutritive value and vitamin content while causing it to contain more pith and hold more water for looks and weight considerations. Growers know this as "the dilution effect." The public attention to the attractiveness of the produce, and its durability in shipping, is considered primary to maximize profits. However, these hybrids are lower in nutrition and are far less effective in protecting the human body against diseases. As told to us in Mitchell:

The adage, 'remember to eat all your veggies,' almost makes no difference here when the broccoli served on your table contains half as much calcium as listed in the 1998 USDA nutrient database.[2]

Add to this the fact that produce is picked green and not allowed to sun-ripen, thereby producing anthocyanins or plant sunscreens which, when consumed, provide the protection that we need against cancer, brain cell deterioration, DNA destruction, and more.

LACK OF MINERALS

The minerals that our bodies depend upon from fruits and vegetables should come from the soil in which they grow, but if this soil suffers from degradation due to erosion or failure to rotate crops, they will not be adequate in our food supply. Soil degradation is not only an American concern but a worldwide concern as well. New farming methods ignore the mulching, manuring, and crop rotation used in the past to restore essential compounds to the soil in favor of chemical fertilizers. Below, we learn from Preventive-Health-Guide.com that:

Historically, these fertilizers, developed from leftover phosphates and nitrates used in the weapons of World War II, were after the discovery that many plants would grow with just three minerals; nitrogen, phosphorus, and potassium (NPK). Thus, the use of traditional farming methods became impractical from an economic standpoint, and the fruits, vegetables, and grains produced from these degraded soils using this new method lack in trace minerals that are also necessary for the body to maintain its optimal health. Although nitrogen, phosphorus, and potassium are abundant in the produce, our bodies continue to become steadily deficient in the other necessary minerals.[3]

FOOD IRRADIATION

Food irradiation remains unproven as safe and is known to cause more harm than good to the foods it is trying to protect. Radiation destroys the vitamin content in produce, but the Center for Food Safety also claims "irradiation forms volatile toxic chemicals such as benzene and toluene, chemicals known or suspected to cause cancer and birth defects."[4] A watchdog group formed in 1971 called "Public Citizen," based in Washington, DC claims, "Public Citizen, a Washington, DC-based watchdog group, charges that the US Food and Drug Admin. has legalized food irradiation while ignoring safety regulations."[5] This further evidence supports a possible link between the FDA's and agriculture industry's common interests:

> The newly released report from Public Citizen and the Cancer Prevention Coalition indicates that FDA's own scientists have dismissed tests used to validate the process. Rather, according to this report, the actual evidence suggests that irradiated food can cause mutations of genetic material and can be toxic.[6]

The long-term effects of food irradiation and how they affect the human body are still unknown. Meanwhile, the Department of Agriculture has announced a partnership with a company in Tennessee to study irradiation and food safety. However, the American public has no choice but to accept food irradiation being dumped upon them all in favor of the agriculture industry whose goal it is to use this process to pursue the more important and profitable global interests of food production.

THOUGH NUTRITIONAL SUPPLEMENTS ARE UNREGULATED, THEY ARE GENERALLY SAFER THAN PRESCRIPTION DRUGS

Accidental overdose from supplements is less likely to be harmful

There are opposing views on this subject and multiple situations to consider in evaluating this. One position to look into would be whether a patient is in the care of a physician treating their symptoms with any medications. If this is the case, the addition of a particular nutritional supplement could magnify that medication's effects and may prove harmful if not cautious. On the other hand, taking the supplement by itself should be safe and non-toxic even if the subject shows to have a particular sensitivity to it.

Prescription Drugs Kill More People Than Nutritional Supplements

In 1994 Consumer Reports sided with FDA approved propaganda by publishing a magazine cover emblazoned with the words, "Dangerous Supplements!" The gist of the article was to substantiate pharmaceutical drugs' safety by referring to them as being well tested and safe while herbs, used over centuries, are dangerous. Adams says, "The article makes absolutely no mention of the 100,000 deaths and more than two million injuries caused by prescription drugs each year.[7] He goes on to state that,

At least 100,000 deaths are caused each year in the United States by prescription drugs, even according to the American Medical Association's own research. Yet the consumption of nutritional supplements can't even be linked to a hundred deaths each year in the United States.[8]

If one does the math, it means that the ratio of death by prescription drugs as compared to by nutritional supplements is 1000 to 1.

Here is a summary of what we now see in our food supply: 1) Prematurely picked fruits and vegetables without minerals; 2) irradiated foods without vitamins that contain toxic substances; 3) the use of hydrogenated fats to preserve shelf life, and 4) flavorings and addictive substances in processed food. There is little doubt that our food supply has succumbed to severe degradation. Many years ago, fruits and vegetables were all organic. Now, with the industrialization of the agricultural industry, premature aging, ill health, disease, and obesity plague many baby boomers and their offspring, thereby fueling a search for organic, healthy foods in addition to quality-controlled nutritional supplements. As public awareness increases over time with information obtained through various communication channels, we now have, especially the Internet, many people are taking responsibility for their health as opposed to leaving it in the hands of doctors alone. Many are aware that the reason a plethora of drugs are available in the marketplace is that the pharmaceutical industry's goal is to treat every symptom and provide temporary relief as opposed to treating the underlying cause for the sign, of which most doctors are ignorant.

As people age, many visit doctors just to complain about what ails them, and the doctor happily dispenses some kind of pill or a prescription and says, "try this." When it comes to your body, choosing chemical experimentation by an unenlightened physician with only a warning of potential side effects may lead to slow suicide. Instead, testing yourself using harmless substances to aid your body's natural ability to fight disease and possibly defeat the underlying cause of your symptoms is the road to take towards better health.

The naturopathic physicians that I continually learn from, and I recommend that everyone supplement 90 essential nutrients. What makes them necessary nutrients is because the body does not manufacture them. However, when consumed and absorbed regularly, the results can be miraculous. These nutrients consist of 60 minerals, 16 vitamins, 12 amino acids, and two essential fatty acids. The conclusion came from thousands of autopsies on humans of varying ages and animals and applied to all vertebrates. Yes, even crocodiles get diabetes!

In your quest to find companies that manufacture quality nutritional supplements, you will discover that all supplements are not of the same potency or quality. The dietary supplement industry is a non-regulated one. Therefore, the quality of the products sold to the public will vary unless they have received the NSF Certification. The NSF certification, which is recognized by regulatory agencies at the local, state, federal, and international levels, demonstrates that a product complies with all standard requirements for safety, quality, and performance.

The "Healthy Paks" by Youngevity that we feature on our website contain all 90 nutrients, and if the 90 nutrients were purchased separately, it would be too expensive for most people to afford. Youngevity products have the NSF Certification. Further, the fish oil has the IFOS Certification ensuring the standard of fish oils is the highest in purity, potency, and freshness.

All the brands we recommend observe strict quality control and are pharmaceutical grade. https://VitalityNowHealth.com carries nutrition that we stand behind because we know the products we sell and have used them for years.

---

1. Mitchell, Terri. (September 2005). Vitamin-less Vegetables. Retrieved November 4, 2008, from http://www.lef.org
2. Mitchell, Terri. (September 2005). Vitamin-less Vegetables. Retrieved November 4, 2008, from http://www.lef.org
3. Preventive-Health-Guide.com. (2008). Is Degradation of the Food Supply The Main Cause of Degenerative Disease? Retrieved November 8, 2008, from http://www.preventive-health-guide.com/degenerative-disease.html
4. Center For Food Safety. (2008). *Food Irradiation*. Retrieved November 9, 2008, from http://www.enterforfoodsafety.org/food_irrad.cfm
5. Center For Food Safety. (2008). *Food Irradiation*. Retrieved November 9, 2008, from http://www.enterforfoodsafety.org/food_irrad.cfm
6. Food Service Director. (Nov 15, 2000). *Watchdog group slams irradiation*. Retrieved November 5, 2008, from GALE Cengage Learning database.
7. Adams, M. (April 13, 2004). *Consumer Reports Article Support FDA's Attempt To Regulate or Outlaw All Nutritional Supplements*. Retrieved November 15, 2008, from http://www.naturalnews.com/z000944.html
8. Adams, M. (April 13, 2004). *Consumer Reports Article Support FDA's Attempt To Regulate or Outlaw All Nutritional Supplements*. Retrieved November 15, 2008, from http://www.naturalnews.com/z000944.html

Chapter Eight

STEP 7: EMBRACE SPIRITUALITY

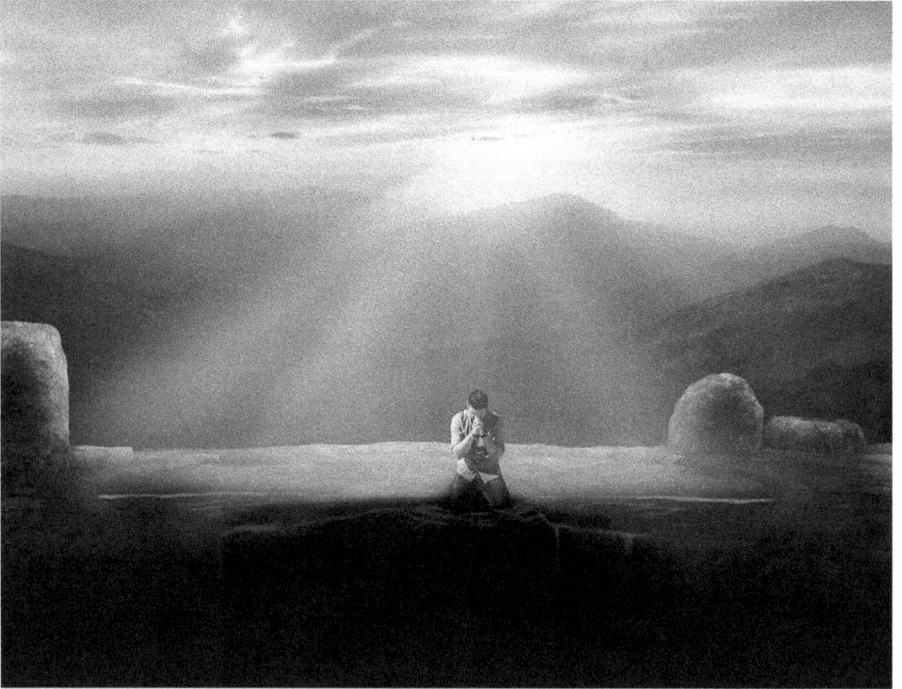

"My son, keep your father's command,

And do not forsake the law of your mother.

Bind them continually upon your heart;

Tie them around your neck.

When you roam, they will lead you;

When you sleep, they will keep you;

And when you awake, they will speak with you.

For the commandment is a lamp,

And the law a light;

Reproofs of instruction are the way of life."

Proverbs 6:20-23

When it comes to spiritual culture, there are both good and bad elements. Today there exists a tendency to balk at tradition and reject the ways of old in favor of newer cult-based religions and philosophies. Most of these views tend to restrict freedom (adding more stress) and never are to be questioned unless one is prepared to be labeled a heretic or infidel, sometimes punishable by beheading. But when you choose to solely accept what is seen by the naked eye as told to us using the myopic vision of science, you miss the bigger picture. The big picture is where spirituality reigns. We are limited by seeing *with* the eye if we do not take the time to see *through* the eye.

The words "religion" and "religious" are not bad words. Religion means to re-align one's self with God. Many people have arguments over what religion is good or bad, but what is more important for humankind is an individual's pursuit of God's knowledge. It is the knowledge of God that increases faith in that which is unseen. Every person is born with a sense of God's higher power and authority. However, the world's systems misshape this natural phenomenon. If an individual does not continually undertake steps for "re-alignment," the student of God will become absorbed by the world's ways and lose their equilibrium. Jesus' parable of the sower in Matthew 13:18-23; Mark 4:13-20; or Luke 8:11-15 are the perfect examples that illustrate this meaning. It is crucial to maintain one's perspective of

God, who represents good concerning the world in which evil is paramount.

It is impossible to sustain the idea of an atheist because it is impossible to prove that God doesn't exist. Likewise, a student of God cannot prove that God indeed exists. So at best, such a person may be labeled as being agnostic. But I ask the question, "Wouldn't it be better to be right in accepting that God exists than to be wrong in asserting that God doesn't exist after considering the consequences?" After all, death's finality is guaranteed, and when it arrives, it will be too late for negotiation.

I believe Jesus would press the atheist to realize the ultimate end of his or her worldview. If there is no God, then our existence is ultimately without meaning, significance or hope. The dilemma facing humankind is that we cannot live in a world where our existence is meaningless, which makes is impossible for atheists to consistently live out the implications of their worldview.[1]

In these uncertain times of chaos, God is indeed the anchor that will help you survive any storm. Never running out of resources, God promises to never leave or forsake you, especially in your darkest hour. I am convinced that it is God's love that gives us the compassion to help others in their time of need, even at the expense of self. Being a disciple of God brings peace in times of trouble, provides many resources, and creates a heart that gratefully shares with others.

---

1. Geisler, N., et al. (2009) The Apologetics of Jesus. Grand Rapids, Michigan. Baker Books P. 127

www.ingramcontent.com/pod-product-compliance
Lightning Source LLC
Chambersburg PA
CBHW051039030426
42336CB00015B/2958